MANAGING YOUR WEIGHT

Why your body may be working ing against you and what you can do about it.

Holly Fourchalk, PhD, DNM®

CHOICES UNLIMITED
FOR
HEALTH & WELLNESS

Choices Unlimited for Health & Wellness
Dr. Holly Fourchalk, Ph.D., DNM®, RHT, HT
Tel: 604.764.5203
Fax: 604.465.7964
Website: www.choicesunlimited.ca
E-mail: holly@choicesunlimited.ca

Editing, Interior Design and Cover Design:
Wendy Dewar Hughes, Summer Bay Press

ISBN: 978-0-9868775-4-4
Digital ISBN: 978-0-9868775-5-1

To my Parents

For all their support and encouragement
My Dad for his ever listening ear
My mother for her open mind

MANAGING YOUR WEIGHT

CONTENTS

ONE

A Short History of Weight Management

As with many issues in life, the perception of the perfect weight has changed tremendously across time and across cultures. Many blame the current media for creating and distorting the perception of health in terms of what the "ideal" body size and shape should be but it is far more complicated than that.

History shows us how hilarious we are – how political, environmental and economic cultures all have an impact on the general public's perception of the ideal female body shape. Today we have taken that a step further. We have added in the influence of the media. In addition to increased print, we have television, movies, internet, and more.

However, throughout history any current ideal of what the female body "should" look like has been difficult to attain. Women are phenomenal. They will sacrifice themselves, i.e., their comfort, their hunger and their health, in attempts to achieve the impossible.

In addition, different cultures throughout history have evolved specific ways of understanding the human experience with respect to what defines a body that is healthy and in balance. Different cultures and different medical beliefs also have different opinions in terms of how and why the body gets out of balance and also how to restore balance.

Who defines balance for your body – the culture, politics, or economics? How does a society determine what is best for all? Who has that power?

To whom do you give that power?

AYURVEDIC MEDICINE

Ayurvedic philosophy identifies three aspects to any component of life. Believed to be the oldest known medicine, Ayurvedic medicine has a philosophy about life, a strategy to live by and an understanding of the human psychology and physiology. It suggests that there are three major aspects to any component of life. For instance, whether we look at:

- How you think
- How you feel
- How you look
- How you behave
- What you desire/avoid
- What you eat/avoid

Old Ayurvedic scripts even describe the cell, molecule, atom, and electron in terms of the balance between these 3 basic components called : Vata, Pitta, Kapha.

These three components, called doshas, each have a very detailed characterization, but briefly could be described as movement, transformation and structure or Vata, Pitta, Kapha.

The balance of these three doshas is unique to each body and the particular balance in your body will determine for you:

- The body shape
- The body functions
- The metabolism
- The disease predisposition

Thus the cause of your weight issue is looked at very comprehensively and without criticism or judgment.

TRADITIONAL CHINESE MEDICNE

In TCM (Traditional Chinese Medicine) the cause of the weight imbalance is looked at primarily in terms of the acupuncture meridians (which were actually determined first by Ayurvedic medicine).

There are 12 parallel meridians with dynamic connections between them. They are assessed predominantly in terms of cold/congestion or a yin condition; or heat/inflammation or a yang condition; and movement (Qi).

For example, the cause of imbalance might be cold/congestion in the stomach/spleen meridian or poor Qi in the Triple Burner, or too much yang in the kidney meridian. These issues would be treated initially by herbs then later, the acupuncture system was developed which was utilized in conjunction with the herbs.

Dealing with these perspectives to bring the body into balance can be very effective.

However, dealing with alternative perspectives on weight management is going way beyond the scope of this book. Just looking at a variety of variables from a Western perspective is going to be extensive enough.

In fact, even looking at the Western perspective and its development over a prolong period of time is going to be beyond the scope of this book.

So let's take a quick look at the social changes and medical perspectives that have occurred in Western society over the past few hundred years.

Prior to the 1900s, society embraced big, buxom, strong women. This body type was considered ideal.

Women with a strong, able body were perceived to be fertile and hardy enough to have greater numbers of children who then helped to take care of the house, the crops, and the elderly. They were also considered robust and healthy enough to work the fields.

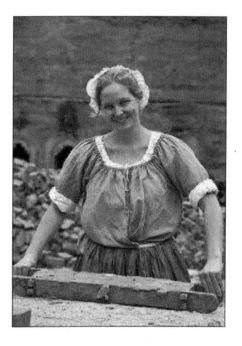

During the 1900s ideas shifted as the need for large families shifted. Women with large chests and tiny waists were considered the most valued. In the upper echelons of society, slaves were bought to do all the chores in and out of the home. The women became "ladies" whose role became to sit around and look pretty. As men were required to do less and less, the women whom they attracted also had to do less and less.

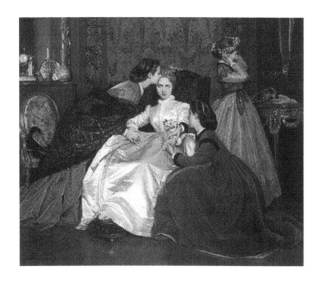

Perhaps because of an age old concept that men needed to take care of women, men were attracted to women who were more "fragile" and less capable of looking after themselves or perhaps the practice developed simply to support the male ego.

This concept of the ideal woman being fragile developed to such an extent that the "fine art of fainting" was taught in finishing schools. To reduce the size of a woman's waist, boned corsets became the vogue, and if the family was wealthy, women would actually have lower ribs removed to further decrease the size of the waist.

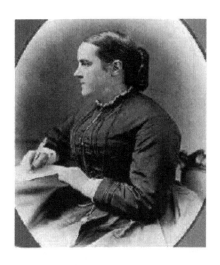

During World War II, women had to go to work and replace the men who had gone overseas. Now women who were strong, competent and capable were appreciated once again. Women became engaged in professional sports and worked in industries and manufacturing plants.

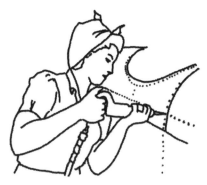

When the men returned home, social perception changed life again. Marriage and families were more valued and men chose women who would provide families for them. Women went back to wearing dresses and skirts and showed off how curvaceous they were, i.e., how capable they were to produce children. Every woman attempted to become like Marilyn Monroe.

The 1960s brought the introduction of oral contraceptives, the renewal of the fight for equality, and values shifted again. Women tried to look more like men and thin, straight, boyish bodies became the look they valued.

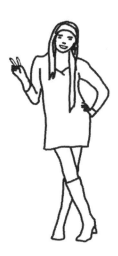

Today we have a totally different situation happening... We are confused about what it is that men want; what women want; and why?

To start with, women wanted to be equal to men and they certainly got it all – household chores, education, careers and looking after the children – the ability to be independent or choose to stay home and raise children or both. Along with all these options came choices in body style, clothing style, etc.

(Unfortunately, while most men liked having women bringing in additional income not all were willing to pick up the slack at home. But that is a whole other book, so let's get back to body styles.)

When it comes to what is today's ideal female body...there is a lot of confusion. Another way of looking at it is that there is a lot of leeway to determine what you want rather than what society says you should want.

With all the media that is present there is a wide variety of ideal body shapes to choose from, such as:

- Thin and emaciated, anorexic
- Thin and undeveloped (upper and lower)
- Full and voluptuous upper but thin lower
- Curvaceous
- Strong and athletic

The four most commonly recognized female body shapes can be compared to the shapes of banana, apple, pear and hourglass. We women can be hilarious whether it is in regard to our hair, our eyes, our body shape or our weight. As a general rule, we are never happy with what we have. We think life will be better when we have what someone else has.

Once you have read through the 4 most common shapes ask yourself:

- what you were born with
- what you have struggled to be
- what it has cost you trying to be something you are not

The Banana shape is straight down without curves, considered by some to be a more masculine shape. Fat is evenly distributed throughout the body.

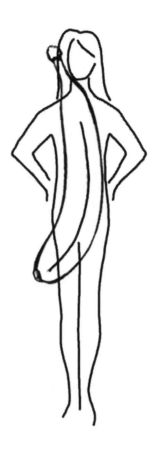

The Apple shape is like a downward triangle with broader shoulders and narrower hips. Women with this body type have slim thighs and legs but have large chest and thick middle.

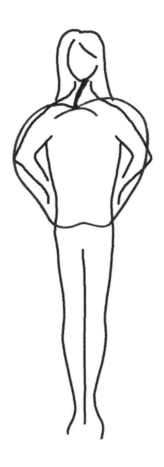

The Pear shape has a larger hip measurement than upper body size. Fat is distributed first to the buttocks, hips and thighs.

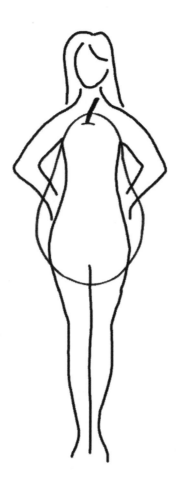

Finally, the Hourglass shape describe those whose hip and breast size have a similar circumference but with a very small waist.

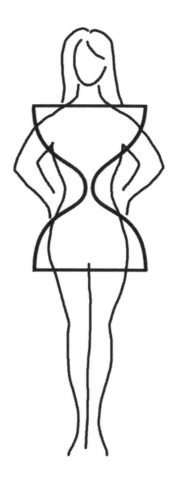

In 2005, North Carolina University completed a study that found that these four body shapes had the following distribution throughout the population:
Banana shape: 46%
Apple shape: 14%
Pear: 20%
Hourglass: 8%

In addition, the study revealed that since the 1950s, waist sizes have increased about 6 inches; women are taller and have bigger chests and hips. However, while women have more options to choose from it has become more difficult to attain the option you want for a wide variety of reasons. Is nothing ever easy?

Increasingly, the challenge of finding good whole food, in the last few decades, has become increasingly more difficult. Food itself has undergone huge changes. Let's look at some of them.

We all know that in today's world problems with overweight and obesity are at epidemic levels. North America is one of the most over-fed and under-nourished cultures in the world, perhaps throughout all history. So with all of this nutrient deficient food and all of the options for body image, what do we do?

Increasingly, the challenge of finding good, whole food in the last few decades is that the food has undergone one or more of the following changes.

Processing

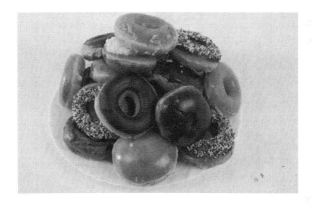

Processing of foods began with pasteurization. Pasteurization involves heating foods to temperatures between 160 – 200 degrees Fahrenheit. This process "de-natures" the nutrients and de-naturing prevents our bodies from recognizing the nutrients or being able to actively engage with them.

Then we started processing meats by

adding sodium nitrates to keep them "nice and red" looking. Following that, microwaving came along which also denatures nutrients at the DNA level.

The food industry then simply came up with artificial snacks with hydrogenated oils, salt (artificial salt!), highly-processed corn syrup, and artificial sweeteners like aspartame.

Because we do not have the enzymes to break these unnatural foods down into molecules the body can utilize, the food becomes toxic.

Toxic Chemicals

Unless your food is certified organic it may have been subjected to one or any of the following chemicals.

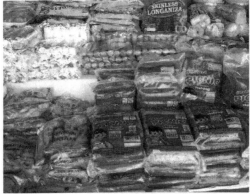

Anti-biotics

It is claimed that 70% of anti-biotics in North America are found in our food supply. Now studies are finding antibiotic resistant bacteria in conventional poultry.

http://www.naturalnews.com/028024_antibiotics_animals.html
http://www.environmentalhealthnews.org/ehs/news/antibiotics-in-crops/

Food colorants – Blue 1 & 2, Red 3, Yellow 6 and others.

Herbicides and growth hormones – such as rBGH in cattle and milk. (This is a problem primarily in U.S. The Canadian dairy industry is highly-regulated.)

Metals – like arsenic in chicken; mercury in fish; lead in drinking water.

Noxious gases – such as those released by Teflon cooking materials.

Organic compounds – that are deadly, like bisphenol-A in the lining of canned foods, polybrominated diphenyl, ethers, polychlorinated biphenyl and dioxins which have been banned but still found in soils.

BPA - Bisphenol A used to harden plastics but leaches into food and water (in the urine of up to 92% of adults).

Flame retardants - in butter.

Mercury - found in farmed fish; destroys the immune system.

Methylnaphythalene - an oil in wax coated food packaging, can leak into food.

PBDE - polybromiated diphenyl ether (fireproofing compound).

PCBs – polychlorinated biphenyls used in electrical and industrial processes. (For a great article found on PCBs visit:

http://www.ewg.org/news/monsanto-hid-decades-pollution-pcbs-drenched-ala-town-no-one-was-ever-told

PFOA - perfluorooctanoic acid, linked to infertility, liver, pancreatic cancers (microwavable popcorn).

PFCs – perfluorochemicals used in non-stick cookware and water repellant food packaging and microwaveable foods (associated with cancer, infertility, high cholesterol and liver problems).

Pesticides, Herbicides and Fungicides (like dioxin and DDT) sprayed onto foods before harvesting; in the ground during production of 70% of conventionally grown foods. (If your potato won't sprout – it is not fit to eat.)

Phthalates: often in dairy products; used in water and soda bottles.

rBGH or rBST - growth hormone injected into cattle (causes breast, prostate & colon cancers).

http://www.ewg.org/healthyhometips/toxi cchemicalsinfood
http://www.lifescript.com/diet-fitness/articles/archive/diet/eat-well/toxic_chemicals_in_food.aspx

Xenoestrogens

Xenoestrogens are hormones that mimic estrogens. Since estrogens are fat storing hormones these fake hormones can wreak havoc with the body.

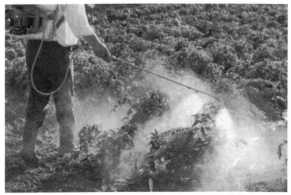

Because we have such a huge additional supply of toxins in our foods *and* we have depleted nutrients to make the body's natural anti-oxidants and other types of detoxifiers, our bodies have no way to deal with all the foreign chemicals and they get stored in our fat cells.

The fat cells, in some areas on the body, begin acting like their own organs and we have further problems.

But let's look, for a moment, at what our foods are lacking.

Food lacking nutrients

Soils have been over-utilized without re-plenishment. In the old cultures, there were various protocols for changing crops; allowing the soil to refurbish itself; usually over 7 period cycles. But today we just use and abuse the soils. We attempt to replace with artificial man made "fertilizers" that do not replenish the nutrients we need in our food.

Recent research suggests that to achieve the nutrient value found in one serving of broccoli from 50 years ago, we would have to eat 20 servings of broccoli today!

Our bodies do not produce the nutrients we need

It is not just our food that is not producing the nutrients we need, but our own bodies no longer make the nutrients we need. For instance, we slather our bodies with sun screens which protect us from the UVB that we need to make vitamin D but doesn't protect us from the harmful UVA rays that we actually need protection from. (There are other nutrients the sunscreen prevents us from making besides Vitamin D, like melanin.)

Without Vitamin D, we do not make...cholesterol sulfates. And why?

We don't allow our bodies to make vitamin D.

Leading scientists now claim that the issue of "too much cholesterol" is not the issue at all; rather we don't make enough cholesterol sulfates.

Another example of nutrient depletion is our rapidly failing capacity to make important nutrients like glutathione (GSH). GSH is one of the most important molecules in every cell in the body.

It is suggested that GSH is involved in more functions than any other molecule in the body. Historically, we lost between 1-2% per year starting at about the age of 20. Now it looks like we are losing between 12-15% per year and starting in our teens!

Product created by man not by nature

One great example of a detrimental manmade product is margarine. It is a synthetic food that was designed to make cattle fatter faster. What's wrong with margarine? It is one molecule away from being a plastic! Yet people willingly spread it on their breads and vegetables, ignorant of what they are eating and how it affects the body.

But wait – there is more

In addition to the problems listed in this very brief outline of food issues we are overwhelmed with stress. Stress causes weight gain. Don't worry we do have solutions. Keep reading.

Our drinking water

We drink way too much water plus our water is acidic and carries all kinds of other toxins. We all know that the molecular structure of water is H20 but those H20 molecules bond together when they are acidic. The more acidic the water is, the more the bonds connect. We will find out more about why this is a problem in the Chapter Six on water.

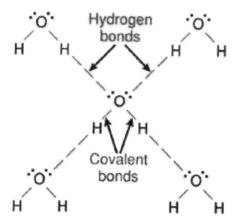

Hydrogen bonding in water.

IMAGE SOURCE: "Chemistry in Context" Wm C Brown Publishers, Dubuque Iowa, 2nd edition, A project of the American Chemical Society, ed: A. Truman Schwartz et al., 1997, Chapter 5 "The Wonder of Water"

Our minds

We all have underlying negative "tapes" going on in our minds. These tapes tell us what we "should do", "ought to do", "need to do", etc., *and* they tell us what we should like. Our minds can change how our bodies functions in a number of different ways. We will get to how that happens and what we can do about it in a few chapters.

To summarize, we have become a society that is over-fed, undernourished, over-weight and diabetic leading to issues of heart health and stroke, arthritis, inflammation, adrenal and/or thyroid depletion, and the list goes on. But if we take the time to learn, we can beat it all. After all we are women.

References:

http://www.independent.co.uk/news/uk/this-britain/the-shape-of-things-to-wear-scientists-identify-how-womens-figures-have-changed-in-50-years-516259.html

http://www.webmd.com/menopause/news/20070820/estrogen-tells-brain-where-fat-goes

http://www.independent.co.uk/news/uk/this-britain/the-shape-of-things-to-wear-scientists-identify-how-womens-figures-have-changed-in-50-years-516259.html

TWO

A Brief Look at Some of the Contributing Factors to Poor Weight Management

As mentioned at the end of Chapter one, there are multiple factors that can contribute to excess weight gain. Let's take a few moments to just review the list briefly. We will then go into each component more fully.

Genetics

You were born with about 25,000 genes. These genes function as off/on switches. Food, thought, emotions, free radicals, toxins, etc can all effect whether these genes turn off or on throughout our lives. We need to turn the effective ones back on again. There isn't a specific chapter on genes, but it is woven throughout several chapters.

Psychology

You live with underlying life themes about how you "should" be. You may have developed coping mechanisms that increase stress molecules in the body that lead to weight gain. Your thinking, feeling, or behaving habits may work for you or against you. Your conscious beliefs may be in conflict with your true self. Do your beliefs come from your family, cultural, social teachings versus your own?

Your stressors, such as how you interpret and respond to the events, relationships, issues in your life may also contribute. Issues in your life may also contribute to weight gain by producing free radicals that end up getting stored in your fat cells. See Chapter 3 for more information.

Fads

Do you shift from diet to diet? We will take a brief look at some of the popular fad diets.

Are you calorie counting? We will look at how ludicrous this whole belief is.

Do you know what really works for you?

Do you know what your body needs?

Are you making losing weight more difficult for yourself? By shifting randomly from fad to fad you actually end up making your situation worse which is one of the reasons many people gain more weight after they finish their diet. But we will look at that, too.

Do you take supplements to make you lose weight or increase your metabolism? Do you even know what that means or entails? See Chapter Three for more information.

Diets

There are so many diets but do you know if they help you lose weight or increase your metabolism? Let's figure it out before you try another one to no avail. Some of these fads focus on elements such as:

- calorie counting
- proteins
- carbs
- fats
- herbs
- supplements
- pH of foods

- preparation of foods

See Chapter Five for more information.

Water intake

- How much is right for your body and how do you know?
- How alkaline should the water be?
- What if it is not alkaline?

What about the Xenoestrogens in plastic containers? Is the water you are drinking actually working against you? See Chapter Six for more information.

Exercise

- Do you need to exercise?
- What is the best kind of exercise?
- What exercise works most effectively for which emotion?

We will take a brief look at all the different exercise programs and the pros and cons of them all. See Chapter 13 for more information.

Detoxification

- What are the controversies about

detoxification?
- What kind of detoxification would work best for you?
- Is your body prepared to detoxify?
- Can detoxification be harmful?

We will provide a brief overview of the different cleansing options, MLM programs, etc. See Chapter Seven for more information.

Leptin and Grehlin

Did you know that most people who have weight issues, either overweight or underweight, have an imbalance between these two hormones?

- Why are these two hormones important?
- What do they do?
- Did you know that most people who have weight issues suffer from an imbalance of these two hormones?
- What do you need to know about them to help weight management?

Another two molecules involved in weight management are adiponectin (a protein involved in regulating glucose and fatty acid breakdown) and cortisol. See Chapter Ten for more information.

Adrenals and Thyroid

The adrenals and thyroid are perhaps the two most important organs for determining overall metabolism. These two organs work in concert with each other. Usually, alternative medicine practitioners, i.e., Drs of Natural Medicine, Herbalists, Naturopathic Doctors, etc. will not treat one without the other.

When it comes to metabolic issues, these organs may work for you or against you. See Chapter Ten for more information.

Muscle metabolism

Good healthy muscles use the greatest amount of calories.

How do you build muscle integrity and not muscle toxicity? See Chapter Ten for more information.

Pre- and Pro- Micro and Macro Biotics

- What do they mean and what do

they do?
- Do I need to be concerned about them?

Enzymes

- How do enzymes impact food metabolism and weight management?
- Do I need to take enzymes and how do I get my body to make enzymes?
- What do I really need to know?

In the following chapters we are going to walk you through each of these components of weight management so you understand:

- the issues
- the controversies
- what you need to do for you

Some will only have to take a few simple steps; some will have to take several steps, but we can all get there effectively. See Chapter Nine for more information.

THREE

Diets and Fads

There are so many diets and fads about weight management it makes me cringe. Let's start with the Weight Watchers routines created back in the 1970s by Brooklyn homemaker Jean Nidetch.

Initially, the "Calorie Theory" was predominantly based on creating a deficit of calories. The belief was, if we ate a shortfall of calories, than the body would utilize stored fats. Thus we would lose weight – sounds good on the surface – but a greater understanding reveals that this theory has a lot of holes in it.

Unfortunately, there wasn't a lot understood about nutrition at that time. For example, there was no understanding of the need for a variety of fats in the body, or of the different mechanisms for different fats. There was no understanding of the difference between Omega 3 and Omega 6 fats and their individual roles in the body.

The problem with the calorie counting system is that it tells you that you are overweight because you eat too much. If that was the case then how come we all know people who are huge eaters and are slim? Yes, intake of calories is a component in weight management but it is only one component out of a huge number of issues.

Today we understand that some calories are good and others are not. For instance, if you spent 1000 calories at a fast food restaurant versus 1000 calories with various organic steamed vegetables, an avocado & shrimp salad, and a baked organic chicken breast your body would respond entirely differently. The following is a brief list of the different impact of whole foods versus fast foods.

Fast Food versus	Whole food
Calories	Calories
Plugs up gut	Helps keep gut healthy
Plugs up liver	Helps feed the liver
Plugs up arteries	Helps to clean the arteries
No nutrients	Bounty of nutrients

Predisposes towards diabetes	Prevents diabetes
Predisposes towards heart disease	Prevents heart disease

Certainly Weight Watchers was not the first fad-type diet but since its introduction we have been subjected to a huge selection of fad diets. Let's briefly review a few of them.

Acai berry Diet

Although the berry is used in conjunction with other foods there is no research to back it. The claim marketed, is that acai berries have the highest ORAC value or the highest level of anti-oxidants. This is wrong. The chocolate seed is now recognized as the most nutrient dense food there is. In fact, it is 2-3 times higher in some of the most powerful anti-oxidants than the acai berry.

While the acai berry does have some important nutritional benefits, more benefit would be derived from consuming a variety of fruits and vegetables. In addition, the amount of polyphenol anti-oxidants from acai that gets to the mouth is very different than what is in the fruit when it initially comes off the tree.

The acai berry diet does not encourage dieters to make lifestyle changes, although like many diets, that is now changing. It supports the idea of a quick fix approach to weight loss and none of the claims have been supported by research.

What the creators of these diets are now starting to acknowledge is simply what others have already been purporting in terms of types of foods and the balance between foods. Unfortunately, like many others, what they are teaching is still a one-size-fits-all kind of approach that never works for everyone.

Three-Day Apple Diet

This diet is based on a finding that eating an apple before each meal broke the weight loss plateau because presumably the fiber makes you feel full faster and you eat less. (This is similar to real chocolate which is full of soluble and non-soluble fibers.)

The Three-Day Apple Diet includes a low intake of carbohydrates and fats; and dieters eat 4-5 meals a day. Apples contain flavonoids that help prevent heart disease, stroke, and some cancers. Meals are balanced with lean proteins, complex carbohydrates, fruit and vegetables.

The problem with this diet is that meals are boring and people quit. It eliminates many foods – some now considered to be important, for example, those containing good fats. This fad diet didn't seem to last long. However, there is an issue with the apple diet that was never addressed. The apples need to be organic.

Most apples are sprayed before they are picked. This gas spray stops enzyme processes in the apples. The apples are then stored in gas bins preventing the enzymes from reactivating. Finally, they are sprayed a third time before being taken from the bins and delivered to the stores. This last spraying re-activates the enzymes so that the apples will now perish if not eaten within a fairly short period of time.

As noted in Chapter 1, these toxins in

and of themselves work against us and not just with weight management but with a number of different health issues.

Cabbage Soup Diet

This plan was a 7-day soup diet aimed at losing weight quickly – which it does because there is a focus on the brassica family of vegetables (cabbage, broccoli, cauliflower). These will help prevent cancers; however it can provoke a lot of intestinal gas, requires good self discipline, is high in salt and lacks good nutrition. Research suggests that most of the weight lost is water.

These foods will help prevent cancers but the diet can provoke a lot of intestinal gas; it requires good self discipline, is high in salt and lacks good nutrition.

Mayo Clinic Diet

Note: there is a fad diet and an official diet. I will address the official one which promotes eating fruit and vegetables, starchy carbohydrates, protein and dairy products.

The diet includes healthy fats like olive oil and nuts, includes whole grains and 3-4 fruits and vegetables daily. It eliminates processed white sugar and limits but does not eliminate meat and low-fat dairy. Like many decent diets, it can work for some; however, there are a number of issues it does NOT take into consideration.

Twelve Steps Raw Food Diet

The claim of this diet is that by eating raw whole foods, the body will get the appropriate nutrients and will lose the appropriate weight. It does encourage a good intake of fruits, vegetables and fats and play a role in a wide variety of health issues. It will certainly reduce various diseases and acknowledges the importance of movement, sleep and too much stress.

It is important to note that according to traditional Chinese medicine too many raw foods can cause stomach/spleen dampness and congestion. This is easily resolved by steaming the vegetables. Steaming activates their own enzymes and this makes it easier for us to digest them. The diet may also lack various nutrients like Vitamin B12, zinc, selenium and protein. Statistics show that vegetarians die younger than the average population.

The creator of this diet claims that cravings for cooked foods are more likely to be related to their addictive nature rather than a true biological need. She created a 12-step to raw foods program to help people overcome their addiction to cooked foods so that they will be able to successfully sustain a raw food diet.

Other fad diets include:
- Green Tea Diet
- Atkins Diet
- California Diet
- Supplements to lose weight

Note: Diets should not be confused with cleanses, as there are major differences. A detox cleanses impurities from one or more systems, i.e., liver, gut, kidneys, etc A detox will certainly aid any need to lose weight.

Some of the challenges encountered with most detox procedures are that they may also:

- Cause you to lose too many minerals.
- Fail to restore your immune system (most is in your gut).
- Fail to balance your leptin/grehlin (often increase the imbalance).
- Fail to re-establish your muscle metabolism (usually break it down).
- Fail to restore the pre/probiotics of the gut.
- Fail to address the underlying psychological subconscious beliefs.

A diet is designed to lose weight but typically does not address the above.

You may lose water and muscle rather than losing the fat you want to lose.

Diets frequently do not address your pH health.

References:

http://www.everydiet.org/diet/mayo-clinic-plan

http://www.everydiet.org/diet/12-steps-to-raw-foods

FOUR

Why Diets Don't Work

There are so many diets and yet they don't really work in the long term. Why is that? People can go on these diets and can lose weight on them. The problem is usually the weight is gained back. Why?

There are a number of reasons why these diets don't work. We have suggested several times that there are many issues to take into consideration when looking at how to manage your weight effectively.

This short outline of issues is presented in alphabetical order, for your convenience.

Adrenal/thyroid
Anti-oxidants
Burdens
Calories
Carbohydrates
Detox
Enzymes
Fats

Fiber
Herbs
Leptin/grehlin
Minerals
Muscle Metabolism
pH Levels
Pre- and Pro-biotics
Proteins
Psyche
Sugars
Water

Which of the diets mentioned above deals with all of these important factors? I am not familiar with any – yet every one of these factors contributes to weight management. Now, you may take a look at this and say, "You have got to be kidding? I can't take care of all of those things. I don't even know what some of them are!"

Don't worry. We will go through each of them briefly and then again in more detail for those of you who want to know more. Either way, you will gain an understanding of what contributes to a long term, effective weight management program for life. We will provide some solutions.

I will present each of the issues briefly for those who don't like long detailed explanations. Then for rest, I have provided a more in depth understanding of each issue in its own chapter.

Some health programs deal with a few of these factors but rarely do programs deal with all of them. Do you know which of these factors is most important to your body and mind? Do you know which program is going to address the issues that you need to address? The extent to which any of the above issues is compromised for you will determine the extent that a given program will work for in a long-term, effective way.

As mentioned earlier, some programs are designed for quick weight loss but do not deal with metabolic correction or weight management effectively in the long term. Some programs are designed to deal with a given component but again not weight management in the long term.

Let's briefly look at each of these factors and then we will go over each in depth to find out how to work with it so that you have long-term, effective weight management for life. This short outline of issues is dealt with in alphabetical order, for your convenience. However, the associated chapters are written in terms of how you might want to address issues. Notice I used the word "might". This is because each body system is different and may require a somewhat different approach. Having said that, all the issues need to be addressed, resolved or eliminated for optimal functioning.

Adrenal/thyroid

These are two of the most important organs that determine the body's metabolic rates. If they are working either too much or too little, they can have a huge impact on weight metabolism. Each has a huge impact on the other and therefore, in alternative medicine, they are usually addressed together. There are lots of factors that need to be addressed here. See Chapter Ten for more information.

Anti-oxidants

Most people have heard of anti-oxidants and know that they are important but do not really know what they do or how. Nor do they know that there are an estimated 18,000 known anti-oxidants and each one responds to different types of free radicals *and* each performs a different set of "other" functions. See Chapter Ten and Appendix 1 for more information.

Burdens
This is more of an European term used for all the different types of parasites, bacteria, viruses, molds, fungi, etc. that should not be in our bodies, or if we require them, only at a minimal level. If they start to dominate our immune system then they cause problems. This may occur in the gastro-intestinal tract (GIT) and elsewhere in the body. See Chapter Seven for more information.

Calories
Calories are one of the oldest and most misunderstood components of Western weight management theories. Calories are fuel and every type of food group takes up a given amount of calories to digest and provides a given amount of fuel in return.

Unfortunately, our society utilized "artificial", "synthetic", "pasteurized", "micro-waved", etc. foods that may be loaded with calories but little or no nutrient value.

Further, how calories are utilized changes from one body to another depending on a wide variety of issues. See Chapter Ten for more information.

Carbohydrates

Carbohydrates are hugely important to our weight management. Our bodies need a variety of carbohydrates. But like other food groups, they can be as detrimental as they can be healthy. We need to know not only how much we need but which ones and from where do we source them. Fad diets tend to reduce the overall amount of carbohydrate intake without taking into account that we need them for a wide variety of functions in the body. See Chapter Ten for more information.

Detoxification

Detoxification is hugely important yet we tend to be more diligent about flushing out our cars and changing the car filters than we are with our bodies. We know that our foods are full of toxins, pesticides and herbicides but how often do we cleanse out our bodies?

How can diets possibly help if we are still putting the nutrients through a system that cannot properly absorb the good stuff and effectively eliminate the bad?

Even in our cars, we try to add the correct type of fuel for the car and we still flush it out with an oil and lube. Think of how much "non-effective fuel" you put in your body. See Chapter Seven on Detox for more information.

Enzymes
Most people do not realize that we have over 10,000 enzymes in our bodies. Further, nothing can happen in our bodies, either breaking down, or building up without enzymes.

Therefore, enzymes become vitally important. Most enzymes, especially in the gut, can only operate when the surrounding environment has a given pH level. We need to understand something about these enzymes and about our pH. See Chapter Nine for more information.

Fats

Fats have been hugely misunderstood. While perhaps the majority of fats in today's food sources are actually bad for us, our bodies do require a number of different types of fats. These necessary fats act as transport systems, fuel, structure and communicators, to name just a few functions. When we simply eliminate all fats from the diets, our bodies suffer and we cannot effectively manage weight. See Chapter Twelve for more information.

Fiber

Did you know that diabetes can start simply because you do not have enough fiber? There are two major categories of fiber in our food: Soluble and nonsoluble. One is important for the bowels and the other is important for the blood glucose uptake in your liver. See Chapter Eleven for more information.

Herbs

Herbs have powerful effects on the body. They have intense nutrient profiles that help the body do a variety of functions: Some detoxify the liver or the intestines or the blood or the lymph; others balance pH throughout the gastrointestinal tract; others are utilized to strengthen organs like the adrenals and thyroid that determine metabolic functioning. See Chapter Fourteen for more information.

Leptin and Grehlin

What are they and why are they important? These are two really important hormones required in food metabolism and when they are addressed properly and effectively they help hugely with weight management. When addressed properly, they also perform a variety of other necessary functions. See Chapter Nine for more information.

Minerals

Minerals, like magnesium, are required for a vast number of processes in the body, including weight management. See Chapter Seven for more information.

Muscle metabolism

Muscles hold onto to various toxins, just like fat cells. Now, while most of us do not want to create big bulky muscle, we do need good metabolizing muscles.

Muscles do utilize a lot of calories. So,

the theory goes: if we have good muscles
that have a high metabolic rate, they will
contribute well to weight management.
But the theory breaks down when we
start looking at both old theory and the
new evidence.

Further, there is another problem. Many
fad diets actually end up breaking down
our muscles. See Chapter Fourteen for
more information.

pH

You have heard of pH many times but do
you know what it means? PH is an inverse equation that determines the
amount of available hydrogen in the
body. If the pH level is high then you
have a low level of hydrogen ions and
the body is alkaline; if the pH is low, you
have a high level of hydrogen ions and
the body is acidic: note the inverse rela-
tionship between pH and hydrogen.

Your body has many different pH levels.
Thus, the pH measurement will depend
on what is being assessed. For instance,
your saliva will be different than your
hair, urine, blood, etc.
As mentioned earlier, the pH level de-

termines the ability of enzymes to function and thus is very important. See Chapter Eight for more information.

Pre- and Pro- Macro and Micro-Biotics

Most people have heard of pre-biotics and pro-biotics. People generally know that they are important but often don't really know the full scoop on them. Briefly, pre-biotics are the mechanisms that regulate the environment in the gut and pro-biotics are the microbes you want to line your gut with. See Chapter Eight for more information.

Proteins

Proteins are incredibly important. We have 22 amino acids – some that our bodies synthesize and some that we need to obtain through our food, called essential amino acids. These amino acids are the basis for over 10,000 enzymes. These enzymes are used to break down our food in our gut; transform the molecules we get from our food; to build up everything from neurotransmitters, to hormones, collagens, anti-oxidants, bone, muscle, hair, skin, etc. So we need to know what kinds of proteins we are eating; what the ratios need to be; how much we need and where we are sourcing them.

Proteins that have been micro waved, pasteurized, and saturated in toxins are detrimental when it comes to managing our weight. See Appendix 2 for more information.

Psyche
This is where the Dr. Phil mentality comes in. Yes, the brain and/or your mind, depending on how you choose to define both; your interpretation of life; your behavioral and emotional responses to the interpretations, and your underlying life themes may all play a huge role in your weight management. They may also play a very minor role. As you can see from this short list, there are lots of factors that come into play when dealing with metabolism and weight management. See Chapter 5 for more information.

Sugars
Sugars, like fats, are hugely misunderstood. The body requires various sugars for a wide variety of functions: to make fuel; to provide intra cellular communicators, and hormone communicators; etc.

On the other hand, the majority of sugars we consume in today's diet are toxic to the body and cause all kinds of problems. We need to incorporate a system that provides us with good healthy sugars. See Chapter 11 for more information.

Supplements
Supplements are necessary in today's world. Why? Our food does not have the nutrient value it did even 50 years ago.

The challenge is that so much of what is out there, in the way of supplements, just gives you expensive bowel movements. So, what is healthy, and what will contribute effectively to our weight management?

Probably 80% of what is out there simply gives you expensive bowel movements. So how do we know what works? What is healthy, and it will contribute effectively to our weight management? See Chapter Thirteen for more information.

Water
People often think that the problem is whether you are drinking too much or

too little water. The 1960s saw a promotion of a false belief, i.e., that you should drink eight 8-ounce cups of water per day. This came to be known as the 8x8 rule. We will look at why this is false. We will also look at why this isn't the only issue with water but why the pH of water is so important. See Chapter Six for more information.

FIVE

The Psychology Behind Weight Management

Now, you might ask why I would focus on the psyche first. Perhaps that is because my primary career for over 20 years was as a psychologist. Or perhaps it is because no matter what we choose to eat, drink, take as supplements, or how we exercise, our mind can be working for us or against us. So let's start with what is most constant.

What goes on in your psyche impacts every aspect of your life. Our underlying life themes are the filtering mechanisms through which we interpret life. An easy way to understand this is to think of looking at life through a pair of glasses that you can never take off.

For instance, if we always wore red-colored glasses, we would learn to interpret and respond to the world in terms of varying shades of red. This world would have both similarities and differences from the person who always wore green lenses and the person who always wore blue lenses.

Our world would be much different than the person who had a distortion in their glasses that made everything look bigger or smaller or off to the left, etc.

With simple colour differences the structures would remain a similar shape just a different colour. With the more dramatic differences, how we identified the structures, described them, talked about them, etc may change significantly. Yet we move around them or engage with them in a similar fashion.

Now let's apply this understanding to a more psychological realm of operating. Think for a moment how you would respond to the world if you understood the world in terms of being guilty. No matter what was said or done, you were somehow guilty.

Now imagine what your life would be like if you interpreted everything that was said or done in terms of never being good enough. How about if you were always afraid, or ashamed, or never heard or were egocentric? We all have primary and secondary underlying themes whether we are aware of them or not. We also have ways of managing these themes that may work for us or against us. These are called coping mechanisms and defense mechanisms.

These themes not only determine how we interpret the world but the coping mechanisms regarding these themes impact on how we respond to the world. And ultimately, the interpretation and the response to the interpretation impact on how effectively we are in our interaction with the world. They determine whether we have an effective perception of ourselves; whether we are effective in our relationships with others; whether we are effective in our careers; etc. These are the components with which therapists usually deal with.

Unfortunately, therapists are not taught how these thoughts and emotions actually impact our adrenal functioning, our internal pH levels, our glutathione levels, etc. Yet, to have good weight management we need to understand whether our underlying themes are affecting all the other functions that affect our weight management.

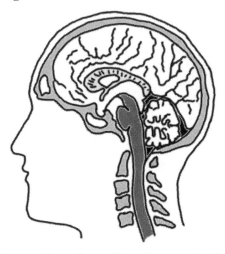

As I mentioned earlier, I practiced as a Registered Psychologist for over 20 years. I was able to read, to study and to listen to a wide number of perspectives from the likes of Dr. Phil to really hard core science. (You can breathe easily, I am not going to burden you with all that stuff – that would take too big a book and probably bore you to death.)

What I am going to do is share some vital pieces with you so you can take a look at yourself – however brief or intense you choose it to be – to see if your weight issues have a psychological component.

Remember, this is being done in the privacy of your own space so there is no point lying to yourself. The more honest you are with who you are, the more you are going to get out of this. So let's start.

Our associations with weight and people and ourselves

We are going to look at several basic questions. When looking at these questions consider two thoughts:

- What were you taught verbally and by whom?
- What was actually modeled to you by behavior and by whom?

Others may be parents/family or friends/others on the playground or teachers/pastors etc. Anybody that you held in high esteem could have had a powerful impact by modeling. Further, even people you held in low esteem might have had an impact on you. For instance, the school or class bully; an abusive parent or sibling; etc.

So remember the directions and let's look at some basic questions:

- What did you learn about appearances as a child?

- Was it important always to look your best?

- Did you have to get dressed up to go out anywhere?

- Were you taught to determine who a person was from the perspective of who they were on the inside or were outside appearances a more important factor?

- Were there different rules for yourself than the rest of your family *or* between yourself and others outside of your family?

- What did you learn about heavy people: Were they lazy; did they eat to more or eat bad diets? Were they of less or more value; did that mean they had money or had no money; did that mean they had great personalities or lousy personalities?

- Were heavy people look up to or frowned down upon?

- Did you have good relationships with heavy people?

- Did they provide you with positive feedback about yourself?

- Were you compared to others who were of greater or lesser weight than you?

- Were those who had a different weight treated differently?

- Did parents, teachers, friends treat you differently than those with greater or lesser weight?

- Were you of more or less importance that those in a different weight category?

- Were people in your kindergarten, primary, elementary, secondary schools, college or university, mocked, criticized or ostracized because of their weight?

- Were people criticized for not looking better than they did? Or for being too obsessive about how they looked?

- Were people ostracized for not looking like everyone else or the "in crowd" or were they valued for being unique and independent?

- Did people with weight issues have great personalities or were they insecure?

- Were people with weight issues fun and entertaining or sullen and withdrawn?

- How were television celebrities, who had weight issues, treated?

- Were television celebrities with weight issues discussed in terms of their performance or in terms of their weight and appearance?

- Were television celebrities with weight issues ridiculed or applauded because of their looks?

- Who did you idealize and try to emulate – and what was their weight issue?

- Were you ridiculed if you tried to emulate one of them?

Now let's jump to the present. There is a variety of reasons people eat that have nothing to do with whether or not their body is telling them they are hungry. After a while these types of associations, beliefs, and behaviors can be become habits. As the old saying goes, "choose your habits wisely."

So let's look at when you eat. Do you eat because:

- You are feeling bored?
- You are feeling angry?
- You are feeling depressed?
- You are feeling afraid?
- You are feeling hurt?
- You are feeling guilty?
- You are feeling worthless?

Do you eat to:

- Celebrate your achievements?
- Mourn your losses?
- Celebrate life's occasions, i.e., birthdays, anniversaries, holidays, etc.?
- Cope with the stressors?
- To protect yourself from relationships?

Do you eat because…

- You are bored?
- You are frustrated?
- You want to avoid something?
- You are lonely?
- You feel ineffective?

With any of the above issues, we can look at what are called "cognitive distortions". Are we dealing with truth and fact or with misconceptions and illusions? This is common amongst anorexics who think they are fat when in fact they are far too thin.

So now let's ask ourselves the following questions: (again number them)

1) Do we have actual data to support our perceptions?

2) Do we minimize or maximize the actual situation?

    a. For instance, do you make a mountain out of a molehill or ignore the mountain?

    b. I gained a pound...but perceive it as if it were 10 pounds? I put on 10 pounds...but perceive is as if it were 1 pound.

3) Do you engage in all or none thinking or behaving?

    a. I am a failure because I ate too much today.

    b. I ate too much for breakfast so I might as well give up

    c. Rather than eat effectively, I go on a starvation diet

        i. Binge or famine style behavior.

    d. Each one of these situations reflects the style of thinking whereby we operate at one end of the continuum or the other rather than finding an effective middle of the road

4) Do you disqualify the positives?

a. When given compliments, are they disqualified or attributed to others

b. This ends up negating the self or reinforcing that the self has no value

5) Do you mislabel?
   a. I cheated on my diet so I am bad, or fat, or lazy, or no good, etc

6) Do you engage in emotional reasoning?
   a. I feel lousy therefore I should spoil myself and eat unhealthy foods
   b. I have a lot of work to do and feel overwhelmed, so I avoid it all and eat

7) Are you an emotional eater?
   a. To get an idea of your emotional eating tendencies look at the statements below and check the statements that are true for you:

____ 1. When I am feeling "down" or "blue" a little snack will lift my mood.

_____ 2. When I'm depressed I have more desire to eat.

_____ 3. If someone disappoints me I want to eat something.

_____ 4. When I am pressured or working under a deadline I have the urge to snack.

_____ 5. I eat more when I am stressed than when I am calm.

_____ 6. If I am worried or afraid of something I tend to eat.

_____ 7. Sometimes when people irritate me I want to get something to eat.

_____ 8. I have had something to eat "just to teach him/her a lesson".

_____ 9. When I get angry, eating will make me feel better.

_____ 10. I look forward to eating something when I'm bored.

_____ 11. I eat more than usual when there is nothing to do.

_____ 12. If time is passing slowly, I look forward to having a snack.

_____ 13. Being alone increases my appetite.

_____ 14. I am less likely to eat when other people are around as I am when I'm by myself.

_____ 15. Eating makes me feel better when I am lonely.

_____ 16. I celebrate with food when I'm in a good mood.
_____ 17. If I'm feeling really good, I don't worry about my diet.
_____ 18. When I'm happy, having a favorite snack makes me feel even better.

Scoring:

These statements are examples of the most common types of emotional eating: depressed eating (items 1 – 3), anxiety/stress eating (4 – 6), angry eating (7 – 9), bored eating (10 – 12), lonely eating (13 – 15), and happy eating (16 – 18).

Reviewing your responses to these statements should give you a general idea of your emotional eating tendencies. Once you know the specifics of your emotional eating habits, you can take steps to address the behavior. You can develop a plan, on how to deal with these emotions in a different way, rather than using food.

Source:
http://www.dredabramson.com/emotional-eating/emotional-eating-questionaire/

These are all issues that you might discuss with a therapist. You may relate to one or more of these issues, underlying themes, etc. You may be working with them and not even be aware of it. If you are aware of it you may have the ability to do the work alone and be effective.

On the other hand, you may need some guidance and support. If you do not know whether you may have any of these issues - or you are aware of one or more but don't know how to deal with them or where they came from then consulting an effective therapist could be a tremendous help.

But as I pointed out, therapists are not taught how our thoughts not only impact on our adrenals and the fight/flight response but also impact on our DNA. Dr. Bruce Lipton's work shows how our thoughts can alter our DNA expression.

If every cell in our body has its own DNA and if the DNA determines what is made and how it is made then we need to take care of our thoughts and make sure they are working for us and not against us.

Dr. Masuru Emoto's work shows how thoughts and language can alter the molecular structure of water – which is now being studied in several universities. While there are various questions concerning the accuracy and validity of Dr. Emoto's work, there is also a lot of substance to it.

The point being that if our bodies are supposed to be between 70-80% water – and there is huge discrepancy in the literature, about what percentage of water we should have – then we need to attend to our thoughts if they can impact on the water in our bodies.

Many universities are now looking at the whole water issue again...water, a simple tetrahedral format of one oxygen and two hydrogens...is the not the simple Newtonian science we used to think it was. Again, considering our bodies, should be between 70-60% water, we need to take a closer look and will do so in Chapter Six.

SIX

There's More to Water than you Thought.

Now most of us have heard that you need water to lose weight; that water flushes out the toxins; that water breaks down the fat, etc. Some of this is true and some is not. So let's correct some of the assumptions first and then we will look at the two most important aspects of water.

The first issue:

Water does not necessarily flush out toxins. We could break down toxins into categories: fat soluble toxins and water soluble toxins. Water can certainly help flush out the water soluble toxins in our bodies through the blood -> kidneys -> urine. However, the fat soluble toxins are a much more difficult category to deal with.

These fat soluble toxins are often man made: food additives, heavy metals, pesticides, plastics, pollutants, preservatives,

POPs. However, they may also be environmental, for instance parasites.

Further, if water has a low pH, the molecular structure of water is too big to even get into cells unless the body breaks it down.

If the lipids (fats) in the body have become oxidized or developed into plaque, water is not going to flush it out.

If our digestive (gut, liver and pancreas) and detoxification pathways (cellular and liver) are not functioning optimally, these toxins will find their way into systems (cardiovascular arteries and vessels); organs (liver, brain) and cells (fat cells and other cells).

When these toxins find their homes in these areas of the body, these are areas where they can be stored indefinitely *and* cause a huge number of problems!

The second issue:

Water does not break down fats. Fat breaks down fat. Try putting some oil in a glass of water. What does it do? It congeals or pulls together and rises to the top. The water doesn't break it down. Water can break down oils only if it is very hot.

So how do fats break down fats in the body? If they are in the gut, we have two options: enzymes and bile salts. A particular category of enzymes called lipases are designed to break down food fats in the gut. The other option is bile salts originally made in the liver; stored in the gall bladder and released from the gall bladder during digestion. These are the most predominant ways of breaking down the fats we eat.

Fat cells throughout the body have to have their membranes broken down in order to release the fat soluble toxins they have stored.

A predominant category of polyphenols are flavonoids. Important categories of flavonoids are called epicatechins and procyandins.

These last two categories (I challenge you to say either them quickly three times – why does science have to be so difficult to pronounce?) are well-known for breaking through the membrane of fat cells, releasing the toxins, *and* becoming a major component of the clean-up crew. If that weren't enough, these phenomenal little molecules also help to change the DNA of fat cells into fatty acids so that they can be utilized as fuel, leaving water and CO_2 as byproducts. And there is a huge amount of them found in REAL chocolate!

Do we need water to lose weight – well, yes and no. We do get lots of water in our foods, i.e., fruits and vegetables, juice, etc. We do need water to function.

When the body is functioning well we lose excess weight. In addition, the water helps the kidneys flush out excess stuff we don't want in our blood. But too much water or water with a low pH can be harmful to our kidneys.

There are two aspects to water we need to look at:

- The pH of water
- The required amount we need to drink

We have heard for a long time that we should drink more water or that we should drink eight 8 ounce glasses of water per day. But was there ever any science behind that? No, there was not.

Dr. Valtin conducted a ten-month review of the scientific literature and historic documents regarding the necessity of drinking eight 8 ounce glasses of water per day. He interviewed medical experts and he looked for any evidence to support these claims and found none.

http://geiselmed.dartmouth.edu/news/200 2_h2/08aug2002_water.shtml/

His major undertaking found that "the universal advice that has made guzzling water a national pastime is more urban myth than medical dogma and appears to lack scientific proof." His search results, published in the American Journal of Physiology, August 8, 2002 said:

No scientific studies were found in support of the 8 x 8 rule. Rather, surveys of food and fluid intake on thousands of adults of both genders — analyses of which have been published in peer-reviewed journals — strongly suggest that such large amounts are not needed because the surveyed persons were presumably healthy and certainly not overtly ill.

This conclusion is supported by published studies showing that caffeinated drinks (and, to a lesser extent, mild alcoholic beverages like beer) may indeed be counted toward the daily total. In addition it is supported by the large body of published experiments that attest to the precision and effectiveness of the osmoregulatory system for maintaining water balance.

Thirst does not mean dehydration any more than hunger means starvation. Science actually reveals that our thirst kicks in when the osmolality of our blood plasma is less than 2%, whereas dehydration begins at osmolaities of 5% and higher.

Dr. Heinz Valtin claimed that, "Osmotic regulation of vasopressin secretion and thirst is so sensitive, quick and accurate that it is hard to imagine that evolutionary development left us with a chronic water deficit that has to be compensated by forcing fluid intake."

http://ajpregu.physiology.org/content/283/5/R993.long

So what does all this water do?

Unfortunately it can be very detrimental for two reasons:
Most of the water people drink has a low pH value and therefore is acidic. When water has a low pH level, it becomes "sticky" and the actual H20 molecules bond together.

With a pH of 5 – the required pH of tap water in North America – approximately 15 – 18 molecules of H20 bind together. This creates a transport mechanism for all kinds of toxins. So not only does the cardio system, the liver and the kidneys have to contend with all that water, but now these systems also have to contend with all the added toxins.

Not only is the water acidic and toxic but it is too big to cross the cellular membrane – the body has to break it down. Of course in breaking it down, the toxins are released.

What we need to do is two things:

Drink good healthy water. Alkalize water before you drink it. Alkalizing water provokes a separation of 0H- and H+. A good healthy system gets rid of the acidic component and holds the alkalizing component. This process also releases the toxins. Not everyone can afford a Kangen® or other water system but you can purchase alkalizing drops in the health food store that will at least bring the water up to a neutral pH of 7.

Drink when the body tells you it is thirsty.

When the body needs something, it will tell us. If we listen appropriately we will respond effectively.

SEVEN

Detoxification

I find it interesting when I hear MDs claim that we do not need to detoxify our bodies. Clearly, they take better care of their vehicles then they do of their health.

Detox happens in two primary places in our bodies: in every cell and in the liver. Let's look at both.

Each cell has a huge number of functions that have toxic byproducts that we need to eliminate from our body. There are a few constantly occurring byproducts we need to eliminate. For example, we are constantly making CO_2 through the bicarbonate buffering system, which is designed to help keep good pH balance in the body. We get rid of the CO_2 through the lungs – we breath in oxygen and we breath out CO_2.

In addition, every time one of those 10,000 enzymes functions, there is a byproduct called a free radical. Now remember, that an enzyme function does not typically happen in isolation. To make a given molecule may require a huge number of steps – each step may require several enzymes. Each enzyme function will produce a free radical.

For instance, sugar is required to make ATP which is the required fuel for every cell in the body. The molecule at the middle of ATP is called Ribose. You cannot supply ATP in either a food or a supplement. Your body has to make ATP inside every cell of the body.

While there are three ways to make ATP in the body; most of it comes through the following steps: First is the glycolysis (10 major steps) which then feeds into the Krebs cycle (11 major steps) which feeds into the electron transfer chain (4 major complexes that involve numerous enzyme steps) all to make 1 ATP molecule.

Now remember you need ATP for 98% of enzyme processes occurring all the time in every cell – that creates a lot of free radical byproducts. Our bodies were designed to take care of these free radicals with anti-oxidants. We make super powerful anti-oxidants in every cell of the body to take care of these free radicals.

If the body is functioning well, the body has enough glutathione, super oxide dismutase, catalase, etc. to deal with these free radicals. But if the body is not functioning at its optimal potential, these free radicals get released from the cells into the lymph system.

If the lymph system is already overloaded, it can modify the free radicals before they end up in the blood or cardio system. The cardio system then transports them to the liver which prepares them to get eliminated through the kidneys into the urine.

Now the liver does over 500 functions and in effect supports every other organ and system in the body. When it gets overloaded with toxins or depleted in vital nutrients like glutathione, then the ability and functions of the liver get compromised and *any* system or organ can start to fail as a result.

So let's briefly walk through the logic and the science here. We fill our bodies with toxins (over 85,000 toxins released into our environment since the onset of the Industrial Revolution and 80% of those are found in our home). Toxins get into our system through:

- The air we breathe
- The fluids we drink
- The foods we eat
- The hygienic products we use
- The makeup we use
- The hair products we use
- The household cleaners
- The drugs we take
- The vaccinations we get
- The clothes we wear

Our bodies were not designed to deal with all of these toxins. We do not have the enzymes to break them down in the liver to get them ready to go out through the kidneys. Our intestines do not have the required weaponry to eliminate them and prevent them from blocking up the pathways that allow nutrition to get from the gut to the liver. In addition, these toxins block up pathways, cause inflammation, cause ulcerations, etc., and we just let them build up year after year.

In addition, when the pH is low and the

gut immune system is also compromised and not functioning at its optimum then many other organisms can take refuge and establish habitat in the gut. For instance, bacteria and viruses are detrimental, as are yeast, molds, tapeworms, etc. These different organisms can cause a variety of issues like weight gain, constipation or diarrhea, leaky gut syndrome, allergies, and more.

Even in the ancient healing arts, before all this extra toxicity flooded our bodies, detoxification was always a component of healing.

In Ayurvedic healing, for instance, the treatments would start off with one of many protocols designed to prepare the body to detox. The second step would involve the detoxification process – again one of many different types of protocol depending on the body's predominant metabolic style and the style of the imbalance. Then the third step was designed to revitalize with various nutrients.

Today, however, we have a much higher requirement for detoxification. But how many people detox? While detoxification has become a component of many weight loss programs, unfortunately, it is often done poorly. Why? One of the reasons is that we tend to lose a lot of minerals with most of the weight loss detoxifications.

In addition, most do not restore the immune system before, during or after the detoxification. This is hugely important and challenging to do. Why? Most of your immune system is in the gut yet products that attempt to help the gut flora tend to drop it all at the beginning of the small intestine.

One company, Qivana®, does have a special patented delivery mechanism that allows different components to be dropped off throughout the gut. This is a very good system.

There are a variety of detox programs out there. Some started out well but have since down- regulated their products so that they are a cheap version of what they used to be. Some started out poorly but succeeded only because they have great marketing strategies. Others are all around good and others are all around poor. Very few are excellent.

Personally, I think the ones that start out as a whole system program are better. These programs involve address the following issues:

- The immune system all the way through the gut
- The adrenal – thyroid functioning
- Muscle metabolism
- Fat cell break down
- Liver and gut detox

Qivana® would be a good example.

EIGHT

pH – What is it and Why is it Important?

pH is an important issue throughout the whole body. As mentioned above, our pH level is an indication of the level of acidity or alkalinity that is in our body. Our bodies are not all one consistent level of pH as some literature indicates rather, there is a wide variation of pH levels depending on what you are assessing.

For instance, the hair, nails, urine, skin, blood all have a different pH optimal level. The gastro-intestinal system has a wide pH variation in it.

The stomach which is not down in your belly but under the heart fluctuates from a pH of 3.5 down to a pH of 1.8. This is where we produce the hydrochloric acid that is the beginning of the protein breakdown. It is also where we create some of our transport mechanisms like the IF that attaches to Vitamin B12 and allows the vitamin to get out of our GI Tract and into our bodies.

By the time our bowel movements make it out the rectum, the pH has to be much higher, i.e., pH = 7 – 7.5 (otherwise it would burn us on the way out.)

Remember, our bodies have over 10,000 enzymes and many of them are in the gut. The challenge with enzymes is that many of them only work in a given pH range. Consequently, even if we have the enzymes they may not function because the pH in that particular region is out of range. If this condition is prolonged, the body simply stops making the enzymes.

However, a healthy diet, provides the body with a healthy pH and allows the enzymes to work effectively.

So we need to take care of this pH just to get the enzymes working which helps us metabolize food properly, absorb what we need to absorb and eliminate what we need to eliminate.

Another important component of the pH equation is that our gut is lined with different bacteria. In school I was taught that there were over 350 different bacteria in the small intestine and over 475 in the large intestine. Yet, since that time I have read of much higher numbers but have not researched the numbers to confirm it.

Regardless, I think it is safe to say, we have lots of different types of bacteria in our gut. These bacteria are called probiotics. But for the probiotics to grow and multiply in a healthy way they need a good environment to live in (called the gut flora) and this is created by the prebiotics.

Did you know that a healthy bowel movement or stool has about 50% bacteria in it? That means that the bacteria have to continually grow and replenish themselves. So it is not just the wide number of bacterias that we require (if you eat really good yogurt without fruit and additives – you get a very small number of the types of bacteria that you require) but also we require a good amount of replenishing bacteria of each type. And as we just said, they need a good environment in which to reproduce in.

Like enzymes, each kind of bacteria can

only flourish if we have the right environment or flora. This flora consists of both the pH level and the food available for the bacteria to feed on and multiply. Do we want them to multiply? Yes. Again, we lose a lot in our bowel movements.

If we are healthy almost half of our bowel movement is bacteria. If we are healthy we should be having as many bowel movements as we had meals the day before and the bowel movement should be about 9" long. That's a lot of bacteria which means they need to grow well.

If we are too acidic due to too much meat, sugar, flour, rice, etc., then the wrong kinds of bacteria flourish in our gut and we also set up our gut (and other parts of the body) to support both the wrong kinds of bacteria and other microbes like yeast, mould, fungi or tapeworms.

Some of these may actually help you lose weight but not in a healthy way. If they rob the body of nutrients, your body is starving. Or they may get bigger and bigger and cause all kinds of other problems as they grow which may put on overall weight even though it isn't you per se.

Some cause problems because of the mycotoxins these creatures excrete. Some gut microbes have a direct correlation with obesity. For instance, a shift in the ratio between Firmicutes and Bacteroidetes can cause one to be lean (a shift towards the bacteroidetes) and if obese (a shift towards the Firmicutes). The Firmicutes also have a positive correlation between loss of energy and weight gain.

(See http://en.wikipedia.org/wiki/Gut_flora)

We call all of these microbes "burdens". Correcting pH, immune balance and doing a detox may correct eliminate the burdens in the system. However, for some, more extensive work needs to be done. For instance, some microbes can handle a wide range of pH and need special immune system activity.

Others may leave eggs that have to be dealt with after the active microbes have been eliminated so that they do not start the cycle all over again. It is important to consult a health practitioner who is well educated in these matters.

NINE

Enzymes and Hormones

A couple of times we have addressed the issue of enzymes in our bodies, i.e., we have over 10,000 and they need to function within a given pH range. However, another important category of molecules in the body are the hormones. Hormones are communicating messengers in the body. They may travel long distances and may cross different systems.

When we are dealing with weight management, the two most important metabolizing hormones in the body are leptin and grehlin. These hormones are well known for telling us we are hungry or full, but will only do so if they are in balance. When in balance they will also do a wide variety of other functions.

Obesity is associated with a lack of leptin but dieting reduces levels of leptin which is one reason why so many diets do not work in the long term. Leptin is made by fat cells and the genes on the 7th chromosome. (The whole issue of genetic disorders will not be addressed in this book, but briefly, you have a genetic disorder it may prevent you from making some required enzymes for food metabolism.)

Leptin tells us we are full by counteracting both neuropeptide Y and anandamide and promoting the synthesis of alpha-MSH which is a long-term appetite suppressant, as opposed to the short term cholecystokinin (CCK), the rapid, "we're full" feeling and PYY3-36, the between meal hunger suppressant.

Leptin is also involved in regulating energy intake and/or expenditure. It is important to the cardiovascular system by promoting angiogenesis (new blood vessels) through the vascular growth hormone. Leptin also plays a role in Polycystic Ovarian Syndrome (PCOS), bone growth, fetal development and bone metabolism. It is increased by perceived emotional stress and estrogen and decreased by testosterone.

Grehlin, on the other hand, is made in the fundus of the stomach and in the epsilon cells of the pancreas. Grehlin increases before meals and decreases afterwards thereby communicating that we are hungry.

Like leptin, grehlin is also involved in a variety of other functions in the body. Grehlin stimulates the growth hormone in the pituitary gland, plays a role in neural metabolism, plays a role in the learning and cognitive processes associated with the hippocampus, plays a role in the nitric oxide pathway, suppresses pro-inflammatory mechanisms in the GI Tract (especially the colon) and increases the motility of the colon (the ability to move the fecal matter through the colon). It is a beneficial component for the regeneration of the mucosal lining of the stomach and some research suggests that grehlin protects the body against stress-induced depression and anxiety.

Adiponectin is another metabolizing hormone. It is secreted by the fat cells into the blood stream. High levels are correlated with low levels of body fat in adults. The hormone suppresses different types of metabolic dysfunctions that play a role in type 2 diabetes, obesity, atherosclerosis, and non-alcoholic fatty liver disease (NAFLD). When coupled with leptin, it totally reverses insulin resistance.

Various polyphenols, like epitcatechin and procyandins, are known to regulate the balance between leptin and grehlin, which again is why real chocolate, is so good for you; thus, eating foods that have epicatechins and procyanidins upregulate and balance leptin and grehlin.

TEN

Adrenal/Thyroid

Many people have heard of hypothyroid but most do not know about adrenal fatigue, never mind what functions the thyroid and the adrenals actually perform.

So let's start with a brief summary of these two organs. We will then look at what they do; why they are connected; and what they have to do with weight management.

The thyroid is important in weight management as it regulates:

- how quickly the body uses energy
- makes proteins
- controls how sensitive or effectively the body responds to hormones

The thyroid is one of the largest endocrine (hormone) glands and is situated in the neck. The thyroid is important in weight management as it regulates how quickly the body uses energy, makes proteins and controls how sensitive or how effectively the body responds to hormones. However, there is a huge misconception about the thyroid and the condition of hypothyroid which is often thought to cause weight issues, particularly in women.

The process of stimulating the thyroid begins in the hypothalamus in the brain which releases TRH (thyroid releasing hormone) which sends a message to the pituitary to release TSH. TSH (thyroid stimulating hormone) stimulates the thyroid to produce T4 and T3 in the follicular cells.

Epithelial cells are usually non-vascularized cells meaning no blood nutrient support. They receive their nutrient through diffusion of substances through what is called the connective tissue. However, they can form clusters that function as glands which are usually very vascularized as they take up nutrients from the blood and release the subsequent hormones into the blood flow.

The epithelial cells of the thyroid take up iodine and amino acids from the blood and make thyroglobulin and thyroperoxidase. These nutrients are released into the thyroid follicules along with iodine. Then with the help of proteases the thyroid follicules make 80% of the T4 and 20% of the T3. The T3 is about four times more powerful than the T4, and about 80% of the T4 – T3 conversion happens in the liver. However, this conversion requires iodinases which can be blocked from action by cortisol secreted from the adrenals. But let's go back to T3 and T4.

T3 and T4 are circulated by the blood, by binding to globulins, to every cell in the body. These hormones cross cell membranes where they bind to receptors in the cells. These hormones regulate the rate of metabolism (conversion of oxygen and calories to energy) and affect the rate of growth and regulate many cellular and systemic functions in the body. Every cell in the body actually depends upon thyroid hormones for these metabolic functions.

When you get a blood analysis on TSH, T4, and T3 you are really looking at the pituitary (production of TSH), the liver (majority of conversion of T4 to T3) and the adrenals (whether or not they are interfering with the enzymes that do the conversion in the liver). What the thyroid is responsible for is the initial production of the T4 and the T3 cells.

Why is this then called hypothyroid? Like most things in the body it is a system process and the body has very dynamic and interactive systems - they all talk with one another; impact on one another; and help to regulate one another.

Likewise when one system is compromised it will also have an impact on the other systems. Another issue is that usually the system has gone through "hyperthyroid" functioning before it ends up in a "hypothyroid" functioning process.

Let's take a brief look at Synthroid, the most common synthetic replacement for the lack of T4. It is not an active hormone. Your doctor, rather than addressing your compromised adrenals and liver gives you an artificial medication hoping the body will convert the T4 to T3.

The challenge is: Synthroid may help

some people in the short term, while they are recovering from stress. However, in the long run it apparently does something else. Under normal conditions your body produces a small amount of rT3 which binds to T3 receptors and prevents absorption of T3 into the cell.

This rT3 isn't a problem unless the body is in a stress response which is usually what caused the hyper-thyroid -> hypo-thyroid issue in the first place. Under the stress response, the cortisol prevents the iodinases from functioning and so there is even less conversion of T4 to T3 in the liver.

Further, cortisol enhances the conversion of the T4 to rT3. So now not only do we have the cortisol working against us but we also have the rT3 working against us. This is called rT3 dominance.

In addition, there is a feedback loop that causes even more of an issue. The Synthroid T4 provokes an excess of the hormone which tells the pituitary not to produce TSH which stops the production of T4 and T3 in the thyroid. Now, with the higher levels of T4 (which is actually just the drug, Synthroid) the body converts the T4 to rT3, which blocks the T3 receptors even further. This ends up causing even more of the original hypothyroid issues than you started with.

So the weight issue is now multiplied and you have been told to stay on Synthroid for the rest of your life – getting worse and worse as the cellular metabolism continues to go down!

You can add to this problem because apparently some of the stressors that have been shown to cause low T3 syndrome or rT3 dominance are:

- Fasting (including repeated weight loss diets)
- Surgery
- Burn trauma
- Alcoholism
- Endotoxin injections
- Clinical glucocorticoids (cortisone shots and prednisone therapy)
- Well that sucks big time – especially if you are trying to lose weight.

Next are the adrenals...these are two glands that sit on top of your kidneys.

Right Adrenal Gland   Left Adrenal Gland

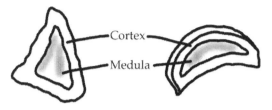

The right one is more of a triangular shaped organ and the left is more of a semilunar shape. The inside component is called the medulla and the outer component is the cortex. Each part synthesizes (produces) and secretes (releases) hormones.

The adrenals are well known for their activity in the flight-fight stress response – when the cortex releases corticosteroids such as cortisol. But the cortex also releases other molecules like hormones, and the medulla releases catecholamines such as epinephrine and norepinephrine (neurotransmitters).

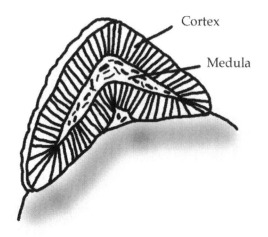

Cortex

Medula

In addition to the flight-fight response, the adrenal cortex also secretes a hormone called aldosterone. This hormone acts predominantly on the kidneys (distal tubules) wherein it regulates the volume of water in the kidneys and thus blood pressure.

The adrenal cortex also secretes androgens like androstenedione (also produced in the gonads) which is required as an intermediate step of producing testosterone, estrone and estradiols (estrogens).

The adrenal cortex has three layers and each layer produces its own hormones:

- The outside layer produces mineral corticoids like aldosterone (blood pressure).

- The middle layer produces the glucocorticoids like cortisol (flight-fight response).

- The inside layer produces androgens like DHEA (required for both testosterone and the estrogens) and a host of other functions that are still controversial.

The adrenal medulla secretes about 20% norephinephrine and 80% epinephrine. The medulla receives direction through the sympathetic nervous system (the activating component of the central nervous system).

What does any of this have to do with weight management? Well, a lot, actually. When one is under stress and produces these corticosteroids, they are difficult to get rid of and it takes a lot of time. In our stressful society, we live on these corticosteroids and depend on them to keep going. The body doesn't get rid of them and they turn into free radicals and/or toxins which end up causing destruction of healthy molecules.

This not only depletes our body's natural anti-oxidants but also the anti-oxidants we take in through our diet and supplements. (Note the body's master anti-oxidant, glutathione, is a million times more powerful than any anti-oxidant you might find in your diet or supplements. It also appears that glutathione is involved in almost all functions in your body whether directly or indirectly.)

However, with the depletion of glutathione, which is increased as a result of the increased corticosteroids, there are even more free radicals. The body protects itself by taking up these free radicals into the body's fat cells. This protection process protects against various different damaging effects but thus the weight gain cycle begins.

The more adrenal cortisol production; the less glutathione; the less able to take care of the resulting free radicals; the more weight gain; the more stress; the more cortisol and on it goes.

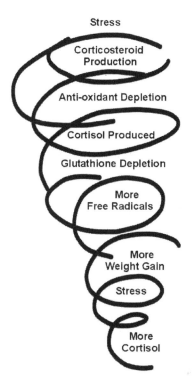

Stress

Corticosteroid Production

Anti-oxidant Depletion

Cortisol Produced

Glutathione Depletion

More Free Radicals

More Weight Gain

Stress

More Cortisol

Important to note that after a period of time adrenal fatigue sets in (although in some situations it may set in very fast) and one needs to be careful. The following symptoms are associated with adrenal fatigue syndrome. See if any apply to you.

- Cravings for salty, fatty, high protein foods, i.e., meat and cheese

- Decreased memory capacity
- Difficulties getting up in the morning
- Feel better suddenly for a brief period after a meal
- Feels better when stress is relieved, i.e., holidays
- High frequency of getting flues, colds and other respiratory diseases
- Increased PMS symptoms such as heavy periods with sudden stops and starts
- Lack of energy in the morning and between 3:00 and 5:00 o'clock in the afternoon
- Lightheaded when rising from a horizontal position
- Often tired between 9-10PM – but resist going to bed
- Pain in the upper back/neck with no explanation
- Reduced sexual drive
- Tendency to gain weight and inability to lose it, especially around the waist
- Use coffee or stimulants to get going in the morning

In addition, other symptoms might include:

- Alternating constipation and diarrhea
- Decreased ability to handle stress
- Dry and thin skin
- Dyspepsia – indigestion
- Food and/or inhalant allergies
- Hypoglycemia
- Increased effort to perform daily tasks
- Lethargy and lack of energy
- Low body temperature
- Mild depression
- Nervousness
- Palpitations
- Unexplained hair loss

At the beginning of this chapter we said that the adrenals and thyroid work in concert and one should not be treated without the other. Let's do a brief summary of why this is so.

Remember that the hypothalamus releases TRH which stimulates the pituitary to release TSH which provokes the thyroid to make 80% T4 and 20% T3. The liver converts about 80% of the T4 to T3, which is 4 times more powerful than T4.

However, if one is stressed, especially for a period of time, the cortisol that the adrenals secrets block the T4 – T3 conversion and allows more rT3 to be made thus blocking the T3 receptors on the cells.

Now cellular metabolism doesn't happen. Conversion of calories and oxygen into energy doesn't happen. In fact, a whole long list of other things does not happen. But the weight gain does happen!

So we need to help strengthen both the adrenals and the thyroid.

References:
http://www.royalrife.com/0103.html
http://en.wikipedia.org/wiki/RT3
http://www.wilsonssyndrome.com/armour
-or-synthroid/

ELEVEN

Sugars – Yes or No?

Sugars have an extremely bad name in today's culture which is both a good thing and a bad thing. Table sugars and high fructose corn syrups are toxic to the body and in particular to the brain. Artificial sweeteners are just as bad and the body doesn't know the difference. We all know about the horror stories of aspartame which has recently developed a new name, (from Nutrasweet to AminoSweet).

Regardless of the name, aspartame in the body still turns into formaldehyde and then into formic acid which is considered the primary mechanism of methanol poisoning. Because of all the controversy and negative publicity about aspartame, it hides behind names like: NutraSweet, Equal, Spoonful, Equal-Measure.

There is a lot of controversy regarding this process in the body but personally I wouldn't touch aspartame in my diet.

The body requires sugar for many processes. For instance, ATP which is the fuel for every cell requires a sugar molecule at the center, called ribose. You cannot supply ATP in either a food or a supplement, your body has to make it inside every cell. There is a long process involved in making ATP that requires a variety of minerals and vitamins like magnesium, Vitamins B1, B2 and B3.

The final component of the process involves the mitochondria and the ETC (Electron Transfer Chain). If you look into a heart muscle – the muscle that never gets to rest – you will find that it requires in excess of 1000 mitochondria in every cell to make enough ATP to supply enough fuel to keep the heart muscle cells going. You need a lot of ribose to make this happen.

Another category of molecules are called glycoproteins which simply means sugar-protein complex. Glycoproteins are required for a number of essential functions in the body, including:

- White blood cell recognition in the immune system

- Platelet aggregation in the blood system
- Sperm-egg interaction
- As structural components of connective tissue, i.e., fibers, ligaments, tendons, hair, nails, etc.
- Found in the mucosa layer of the digestive tracts preventing the breakdown of the lining from digestive enzymes.
- Also found in the mucosa lining of the respiratory tract from the nose down through the lungs

Several hormones are also glycoproteins, i.e., FSH, TSH, etc. There is a variety of different sugars required to make all these different glycoproteins.

The following is a list taken from wikipedia.org and gives a nice chart showing the different sugars the body requires to make these molecules.

There is a variety of different sugars required to make all these different glycoproteins.

The principal sugars found in human gly-coproteins.

Sugar	Type	Abbreviation
β-D-Glucose	Hexose	Glc
β-D-Galactose	Hexose	Gal
β-D-Mannose	Hexose	Man
α-L-Fucose	Deoxyhexose	Fuc
N-Acetylgalactosamine	Aminohexose	GalNAc
N-Acetylglucosamine	Aminohexose	GlcNAc
N-Acetylneuraminic acid	Aminononulosonic acid(Sialic acid)	NeuNAc
Xylose	Pentose	Xyl

Source:
http://en.wikipedia.org/wiki/Glycoprotein

So while the body does not require any of the man-made/man-processed/man-interfered-with sugars, it does require natural whole sugars found in nature.

These sugars may already be in a sugar form or they may be broken down from carbohydrates and redesigned into a pseudo-sugar.

TWELVE

Fats – Yes or No?

Fats are like sugars to the degree that the answer as to whether or not we need them is both yes and no. If you understand the answer then you will know which ones to choose.

Fats, like sugars, play important roles in the body. The liver makes about 80% of our cholesterols (which are fats) which are not only used for transport systems but also for:

- Important structural components of cell membranes
- The manufacturing of bile (used to break down fats in the intestines)
- To make steroid hormones (like testosterone and estrogens) and vitamins (like Vitamin D)

Other important uses for fats in the body include:

- Insulation on the axon of neurons (without it, we develop Multiple

Sclerosis).

- Many vitamins are fat soluble, meaning they can only be digested, absorbed and transported in conjunction with fats.
- Fatty acids are another important group of molecules in the body, i.e., Omega 3 fatty acids are anti-inflammatory.
- Fats are also an energy reserve. When we have no more sugars to make fuel, we can utilize stored fats.
- Fats play an important role in healthy skin and hair.
- Fat cells are also buffers against a wide number of diseases – fat cells absorb all kinds of toxins that the body cannot get rid of because the body is too toxic; or the body is overwhelmed; or the body is already compromised.
- Fat cells also produce a number of different hormones and molecules, i.e., leptin and cytokines.

One of the reasons fats got such a bad name was that old medical science didn't know the difference between Omega 3 and Omega 6 kinds of fats. It didn't know the problems that trans fats or unsaturated fats could cause. For instance, the medical sciences didn't know that the trans fats from hydrogenated oils are far more harmful than naturally occurring oils, or that Omega 3 fats are well utilized by the body *and* are an excellent source of natural anti-inflammatories.

Fats from fast foods and junk foods can cause:
- Coronary heart disease
- Alzheimer's disease
- Cancer
- Diabetes
- Liver dysfunction
- Obesity
- Major Depressive Disorder

In contrast, healthy fats come from avocados and Xocai® chocolate (Xocai® chocolate has a special patent that protects the nutrients found in chocolate including the powerful anti-oxidants and the fatty acids).

The brain requires various different types of fatty acids for structure, for fuel, and for transport. The body requires the Omega 3 anti-inflammatory fats for all the anti-inflammatory processes and we can get all of this in REAL CHOCO-LATE!

Here is a simple chart that will make it easy for you:

GOOD FATS

Monounsaturated Fat
Olive oil
Sunflower oil
Peanut oil
Sesame oil
Avocados
Olives
Nuts (almonds, peanuts, macadamia nuts, hazelnuts, pecans, cashews)
Peanut butter

Polyunsaturated Fat
Soybean oil
Corn oil
Safflower oil
Walnuts
Sunflower, sesame, and pumpkin seeds
Flaxseed
Fatty fish (salmon, tuna, mackerel, her-ring, trout, sardines)
Soymilk

Tofu

BAD FATS

Saturated Fat
High-fat cuts of meat (beef, lamb, pork)
Chicken with the skin
Whole-fat dairy products (milk and cream)
Butter
Cheese
Ice cream
Palm and coconut oil
Lard

Trans Fat
Commercially-baked pastries, cookies, doughnuts, muffins, cakes, pizza dough
Packaged snack foods (crackers, microwave popcorn, chips)
Stick margarine
Vegetable shortening
Fried foods (French fries, fried chicken, chicken nuggets, breaded fish)
Candy bars

References:

http://www.helpguide.org/life/healthy_die t_fats.htm

http://en.wikipedia.org/wiki/Trans-fats#Health_risks
http://www.helpguide.org/life/healthy_diet_fats.htm

THIRTEEN

Supplements

There is a huge challenge with supplements in the health food industry. Many just provide you with expensive bowel movements.

For instance, in laboratories it is easier and cheaper to make mirror images or chiral. We do not make the mirror image enzymes and so these molecules become useless at best and toxic at worse, to the body.

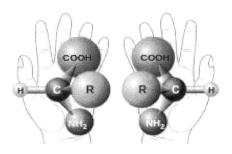

In addition to chirals, there is a variety of isomers – two distinct molecules with the same chemical formula, i.e. all the same components just arranged differently – but then we don't have the enzymes again.

Other types of restructuring involve just reversing two molecules on either side of a carbon structure' or a rotation of a given aspect or plane of the molecule. Although a given molecule has all the same components, there is a variety of ways to change the arrangement. When the molecules are rearranged, we no longer have enzymes that will metabolize them. Then we lose the nutrients or they become toxic to us.

Another problem with supplements is that they are not always what they claim to be. For instance, Vitamin D3 is often up to 70-80% Vitamin D2.

Another challenge is when we have synthetics, i.e. Vitamin C versus ascorbic acid. Real Vitamin C found in whole foods contains:

- Rutin
- Bioflavonoids (vitamin P)
- Factor K
- Factor J
- Factor P

- Tyrosinase
- Ascorbinogen
- Ascorbic Acid

Whereas when ascorbic acid is made in a manufacturing plant, they make the outer ring that serves as a protective shell for the entire Vitamin C complex. Consequently, ascorbic acid does not provide the same benefits as true Vitamin C does. The whole Vitamin C complex will provide the following benefits:

- Helps to form collagen, which is a key structural component of your bones, ligaments, tendons, and blood vessels
- Acts as a powerful antioxidant, protecting your cells against damage and premature aging due to free radicals, toxins, and other harmful substances that make their way into your blood
- Prevents damage to fatty acids, amino acids, and glucose in your blood
- Helps to make norepinephrine, a hormone that is essential to the health of your nervous system

The following are good sources of Vitamin C according to: Dr. Ben Kim who writes about Vitamin C and its derivatives and benefits.

Whole Food Sources	Serving	Vitamin C (mg)
Sweet red pepper	1/2 cup, raw	141
Strawberries	1 cup	82
Orange	1 medium	70
Brussels sprouts	1/2 cup	68
Broccoli, cooked	1/2 cup	58
Collard greens, cooked	1/2 cup	44
Grapefruit	1/2 medium	44
Cantaloupe	1/4 medium	32
Cabbage, cooked	1/2 cup	24
Tomato	1 medium	23

Another challenge with supplements is that they have stearates in them. These are used in the last step of processing.

Stearates are used to keep the machinery in tip top shape and to make it easier to form the product. However, nutritional scientists claim that they are both toxic to the body and they prevent absorption up to 80% which means you are basically paying for expensive bowel movements.

One issue that we mentioned earlier is with glutathione (GSH), a hugely important molecule in the body that is involved in most processes in the entire system. We desperately need this molecule and unfortunately most of us are deficient. We can buy GSH in the health food store and they will tell you it is the Master Anti-oxidant.

That sounds good *but* there is no transport mechanism to get GSH into the cell, even if made it through the hydrochloric acid of the stomach. We are getting expensive bowel movements. Further, the glutathione complex actually involves 8 different components.

If we go to MLMs, there is a huge disparity in these companies' claims. For example, one is known to increase the body's capacity to make GSH 15-30% within a few months versus another, for the same price that will increase the levels of GSH by 300% within one month.

The manner in which the body achieves

these increases is also entirely different but who out there is explaining this to you?

In addition, there is a wide number of foods and supplements that support GSH, although do not provoke the body to synthesize it. So again, you need to consult someone who knows the research.

Another challenge with a lot of products out there is that they claim of have scientific research. Unfortunately, the research may all be "in house", poorly designed, ineffective, or they may be backed by MDs/NDs or celebrities who are paid to endorse the products.

While most in the alternative health field would like these products to be regulated, everyone is definitely against the pharmaceutical companies having any role in the regulation processes.

While these are only a few of the challenges we confront with the "health food industry", you can see why it is important to consult with someone who knows what he or she is talking about.

Typically, it is neither your MD nor your health food store consultant.

FOURTEEN

Muscle Metabolism –
Do I have to exercise?

Muscle metabolism is a huge component in weight management. This is where the gyms make their money. But do you have to get passionate about exercise in order to increase muscle metabolism? Maybe not but being a couch potato is not going to be a strategy for health. Let's explore both sides of the coin.

Imagine a swamp without much movement. The fish are going to die and it is going to get overburdened with moss, molds, and the like. This is indicative of the body that is overwhelmed with toxins and just gets more and more plugged up. This is not a healthy process for the body and more like the couch potato.

On the other hand, having a waterfall of activity or a very fast moving river is also not what we want because there is no opportunity for healthy absorption and metabolism.

As usual, the body wants something that is more middle-of-the-road. We need movement to keep the blood and the lymph and the cerebral spinal fluid and all the water in the body flowing well. This may only require regular walking.

However, we have to look after muscle metabolism as well. Why? Because good muscle utilizes a lot more calories which in turn helps us stay slim.

According to Adam Zickerman, author of Power of 10: The Once-a-Week Slow Motion Fitness Revolution, "three extra pounds of lean muscle burns about 10,000 extra calories a month".

Zickerman also says that three extra pounds of muscle "burns as many calories as running 25 miles a week, or doing 25 aerobic workouts a month without leaving your couch."

However, what research reveals is that muscle actually has a very low metabolic rate when it is at rest, i.e., when you are sitting in front of the computer, your book, or the television. In fact, if you look below, the metabolic rate of muscle is a lot lower than many other parts of the body.

Organ or tissue	Daily metabolic rate
Adipose (fat)	2 calories per pound
Muscle	6 calories per pound
Liver	91 calories per pound
Brain	109 calories per pound
Heart	200 calories per pound
Kidneys	200 calories per pound

http://muscleevo.net/muscle-metabo-lism/?sms_ss=facebook&at_xt=4dbbc2565a2 fec07%2C0

It isn't surprising that the heart is at the top of the list, but most people are surprised to learn that the kidneys are at the top as well with 200 calories per pound. The brain (109 calories per pound) and liver (91 calories per pound) also have high values, personally, that ticks me off. Since I spend a lot of time working with analysis and research I would like my brain to be at the top of the list – not half way down! However, look at how far down the list muscle is and certainly not far above fat.

Despite skeletal muscle and fat taking up the two largest components of our bodies their contribution to resting energy expenditure is smaller than that of organs. The vast majority of the resting energy expenditure of your body comes from organs such as liver, kidneys, heart, and brain, which account for only 5% to 6% of your weight.

So should we just sit on the couch and not worry about it? NO!

There is a major difference in muscle metabolism when you figure in resistance, breakdown, and recovery. In fact, resistance training will accelerate protein turnover thus increasing calorie expenditure for hours, perhaps even days.

Further, after a workout, the body has to get your levels back to normal, i.e., glucose, fats, proteins, etc. It has to rebuild what you broke down; repair the damage from free radicals, and more. I am sure that those with more muscle and more muscle breakdown will burn more calories.

However, if we exercise too much,

whether at a given time or across time, we can end up with lactic acid build up, glutathione depletion and an enlarged left ventricle in the heart.

So what to do? Personally, I walk a few miles with my dogs every day. I make sure I get up from the computer every hour and play with the dogs, do housework or stretch to keep the body moving and healthy, and I engage in my yoga.

I do push not push my clients to pay for a gym membership. I do not push them to go in and work past a sweat, doing exercise that puts them at risk of injury or at a level that accumulates lactic acid, depletes glutathione or enlarges the left ventricle in the heart.

Rather, I suggest steady focused exercise like Pilates or yoga or Tai Chi, going out and getting fresh air by walking or working in the yard. All of these are healthy, effective and good for you.

Two types of exercise that are now well recognized to promote health, good metabolism and weight loss are: Dr. Sears' PACE program or the HIT (High Intensity Training) program. Very simply, both promote pushing as hard as you can for about 90 seconds and then slowing right down and allowing the body to re-stabilize. You work up to between 5-7 cycles and repeat 2-3 times a week – beautiful results without all the negative consequences and risks.

Another method you might want to try utilizing is the vibrational machine. There are many different types out there and they all claim different results but basically they allow people to take a few minutes a week and stand on a machine that will vibrate the entire body at different frequencies to:

1) detox the fat cells
2) detox and strengthen the muscles
3) detox the cardiovascular system
4) detox the central nervous system.

References:
http://muscleevo.net/muscle-metabo-lism/?sms_ss=facebook&at_xt=4dbbc2565a2fec07%2C0

FIFTEEN

Summary

So many issues, what do you do?

Well, here are a few simple sugges-
tions…

Start with a good detox or a cleanse program. My recommendation would be
products by a company called Qivana®.
Qivana® is a good start to a detox, increased muscle metabolism, adrenal –
thyroid balance, good pH and a good
immune system in your gut

Another option you might consider is
Xocai® chocolate. One woman I know
lost 127 pounds in seven and a half
months just by adding the Xocai® chocolate to her diet. Xocai® was the only
company asked to present at the last
Bariatrics Conference and was highlight-
ed in the journal. This cleanse is a lot
milder than some others as the polyphenols (epicatechins and procynandins) release toxins from fat cells and turn the
DNA of fat cells into fatty acids for fuel.

Polyphenols also regulate leptin and grehlin. Xocai® works wonderfully well for diabetics some of whom have eliminated their need for medications and insulin.

Make sure you have good pH levels. Check your urine with litmus paper both before and after your cleanse. You may need to add some alkalizing minerals and/or herbs. Some herbs will increase alkalinity whereas others are known to regulate the alkalinity to what the body requires in a given area. One should consult with an alternative practitioner to understand how to use these herbs effectively.

Work with alkalizing water and alkalizing foods.

Psyche
Work with a therapist to determine if you have any underlying life themes, or negative tapes, with regard to your weight, appearance, safety, what you deserve, etc.

Fats and sugars
Make sure you get some of both BUT

make sure they are the healthy kind.

Vitamins and Minerals
Get an understanding of what vitamins and minerals you need. Find a good knowledgeable practitioner who can identify high quality products, without stearates, that are useful and not simply creating expensive bowel movements.

Water
Make sure you drink good alkalized water. Drink when you are thirsty.

Exercise
Movement is hugely important – even if it is just walking.

APPENDIX 1

Did you know?

Chocolate comes from a fruit called co-coa.

Chocolate comes from the seed of the co-coa fruit and, like most seeds, is the most nutrient dense food there is.

Chocolate has over 300 nutrients the body requires. Chocolate is the number one source of magnesium (and other al-kalizing minerals).

Xocai® Chocolate* is the only company that has a patent that protects all the nu-trients in the chocolate so that what is in the seed gets to your mouth.

Xocai® chocolate significantly improves vasodilation (ability for arteries to con-tract and expand) thus reducing hyper-tension.

Xocai® chocolate has a huge impact on Type II diabetes. I recommend it to all my diabetic clients and they are doing great.

Other types of "bitter" or "dark" chocolate go through "Dutch pressing" and then remove all the fatty acids (cocoa butter). This cocoa butter is sold at a high price for the high end "white chocolate". Unfortunately, this process eliminates up to 80% of the precious antioxidants found in chocolate.

Xocai® Chocolate was the only company asked to present at the Bariactrics Conference November 2011 and was featured in their journal.

3 pieces of Xocai® chocolate = 12 servings of fruit and vegetables in antioxidants alone.

Xocai® chocolate has 19 amino acids – everything your body needs to make the neurotransmitters.

Xocai® chocolate has natural MAOIs which are anti-depressants.

Xocai® chocolate has neurotransmitters, anandamide (blissful neurotransmitter).

Xocai® chocolate has three times the anti-oxidants of acai berry and twenty times the anti-oxidants of green tea.

For more information on Xocai®: http://mxi.myvoffice.com/drholly/

*This information is provided for general information only, and is not a substitute for the medical advice of your own doctor or other health care professional. Always consult your own health care practitioner.

APPENDIX 2

Did you know?

QIVANA®* doesn't focus on the weight loss but rather on reestablishing the metabolic system in the body.

QIVANA® works with systems and not with individual products.

QIVANA® makes a shake that increases muscle metabolism due to its particular ratio of amino acids.

QIVANA® has a patented delivery system that allows for delivery of immune nutrients to each part of the gastrointestinal tract and not just at the beginning of the small intestine, i.e., the duodenum.

QIVANA® has special rights to a herb referred to as King's Crown, GP, or Gynostemma Pentaphyllum. This herb is an awesome adaptogen and anti-oxidant and GP strengthens the adrenal/thyroid organs.

For more information on QIVANA®:
http://drholly.myqivana.com/

*This information is provided for general information only, and is not a substitute for the medical advice of your own doctor or other health care professional. Always consult your own health care practitioner.

APPENDIX 3

Sources for Products

OGF® Original Glutathione Formula

Glutathione is not only the body's Master Anti-oxidant, a million times more powerful than a supplement or food anti-oxidant, BUT, is involved in almost all functions and processes in the body. OGF® is a natural product formulation that provides each cell with a "pancake mix" so to speak, to make glutathione. All the nutrients the cells require to make glutathione are contained in the capsule.
http://www.robkellermd.com/?a_aid=78818

Protandim®

Turns on the "surivival mechanism" genes in our DNA that control: Anti-inflammatory; anti-oxidant; and anti-fibrosis pathways. It also turns on the genes that provide the "tools" to make glutathione.
http://www.mylifevantage.com/drholly/

Xocai® Chocolate

The US Government provided certification that Xocai® is the only chocolate allowed to call itself the "Healthy Chocolate". Xocai® protects all the important fatty acids and anti-oxidants in chocolate in addition to the over 300 nutrients in chocolate.

http://www.choicesunlimited.ca/xocai

Qivana®
METABOLIQ (R) registered r, the only scientifically engineered and clinically proven Metabolic Correction System. It detoxifies the body and improves the immune function of the gut with a patented delivery system of probiotics and a special ratio of amino acids that improves the muscle metabolism.

http://www.choicesunlimited.ca/content/qivana

93199141R00091

Made in the USA
Columbia, SC
06 April 2018